Survival Guide:

Best Survival Lessons on Building Your Own Shelter To Stand up a Storm

Table of content

Introduction

Shelters are necessary to provide protection against the harsh weathers in the wild. Also, they serve as a first defense against the enemies as you can hide inside and wait for the right moment to attack, if necessary. Picking up a location for your campsite is a critical decision not only for the security purposes but self-reliance opportunities as well.

There are many methods and techniques through which you can build shelters robust enough to stand a storm. Camouflaging your shelter is pertinent. It not only provides you protection from the wild animals but also helps you hide your location from the unfriendly strangers.

You can also build shelters in snow. They are made to create an insulating environment for your survival under harsh and cold weather conditions. These shelters can maintain a constant temperature of 36 degrees centigrade. Lighting a tea candle take it up to 40 degrees inside.

You can build your temporary accommodation on a mountain too. But you must consider the risk factors and self-reliance opportunities before constructing one.

Chapter 01: Tips to Select a Mountain to Build Your Shelter

Picking up a location for your campsite is a critical decision not only for the security purposes but self-reliance opportunities as well. Mountains are preferred over other sites because natural water resources are readily available there and also, more possibilities of self-defense are available. Here, we are discussing a few important tips to select a mountain to build your shelter. Let's read together;

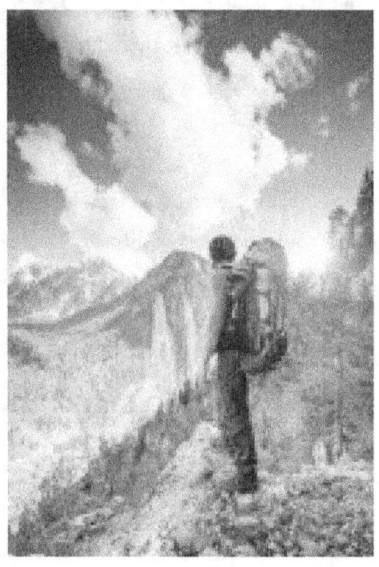

http://i.istockimg.com/file_thumbview_approve/75505359/3/stock-photo-75505359-young-man-traveler-with-backpack-relaxing-outdoor.jpg

Location Distance to the Mountain:

There are two primary aspects of your campsite at the mountain in figuring out the location distance:

1. The entire traveling distance of the campsite

2. The distance between your campsite and the first dense population

Keeping traveling distance of your campsite location as short as possible is pertinent. The further you will take to reach your campsite location from your current home, the more problems you are going to face in the way such as roadblock set ups within hours.

If you are walking to your campsite at the mountain from your current home, then it must be less than a five days distance. One day travel must not exceed 12 miles. It means that the overall distance from the location of the campsite at the mountain must not more than sixty miles away from your current home.

If you are driving to your campsite at the mountain from your current home, then it must not be farther than where one tank of fuel can take you. Getting long-term reliable fuel storage is pertinent if you are planning to go farther than one fuel tank distance. No matter how much fuel you store, it is never advisable to set your campsite farther than a fuel tank distance from your current home.

The second aspect in figuring out the location distance of your campsite at the mountain is its proximity to high-density population.

Your checklist must include:

- Figuring out the distance to check if you can travel between your current home and the desired campsite location within five days on the walk and within a fuel tank while driving.

- Checking if the campsite you want on the mountain is present at a fair distance from the nearest high-density population.

Water Availability at the Mountain:

It is ideal to have a natural water source near your campsite on the mountain. It is not possible to survive without water for quite a long time, therefore, having access to natural water resources like a stream, river, lake, or pond at such sites is pertinent.

Otherwise, you need to have self-replenishing massive water storage system. It consists of rainwater storage systems and large storage tanks.

Abundant water can go way beyond just hydrating you. You can use it for sanitation. You can harness energy through a consistent power generation system on it as well.

You can quickly set-up a hydro-power generation system if you have running water nearby your campsite on the mountain that falls a slope at a decent speed.

Your check list must include:

- What are the nearby fresh water resources at the campsite location on the mountain?

- How reliable are those resources?

- How far are they exactly from the campsite?

- Bonus point: if the water supply is high enough to have kinetic energy?

Securing and Concealing Your Mountain:

After checking the distance of your campsite location from the high-density population, securing and hiding it is pertinent. Unfriendly people may locate you if you are not careful enough. You have found the site, so there is a fair chance for other people to discover it too.

Find locations that are not near to the mountain pass or traveling paths. People go on these routes more often. They can locate you and your campsite. Find locations that are not near to the mountain pass or traveling paths. People travel on these paths more often. They can easily locate you and your campsite.

After finding one good location, you need to conceal your tent, RV, shelter or cabin on it. A camouflaged location is not easy to find. Also, wanderers cannot see you from a distance.

Also, check if the smoke and scent, when you heat or cook, will attract people to your location or not. It is ideal to contain your fire during the daytime and light it at night only. It will hide the smoke.

Another important thing is to check that how many people are using the natural water resource that you have located for your use. Too many people coming there is not okay for your campsite.

Your checklist must include:

- How can you camouflage your location and tent?

- If people can detect smoke and scent of your cooking and heating from a fair distance?

- How much populated is the nearby natural water resource?

Self-Reliance Opportunities at Your Mountain:

We have discussed hydro-power generation earlier. If you are camping in an area with a lot of sunlight, then you can check out the solar power generating ideas as well.

Also, test the food-producing potential of soil around your campsite. If the mountain is all rocks and no soil then growing a vegetable garden, there is going to be a challenge for you.

You will also need abundant firewood around your campsite. Therefore, too much rocky area with no trees does not suit you.

You may also plan to raise some livestock on the location for food. Check if there is enough grass to feed them. You may also need to grow food to support your chickens.

Your checklist must include:

- Is there enough sunlight to install a solar panel for power generation?

- What is the food-producing potential of the soil around your campsite?

- Does the area contain abundant firewood?

- Can you raise livestock at the campsite or not?

Chapter 02: Half-cave and Fallen Tree Shelter

Shelters are necessary to provide protection against the harsh weathers in the wild. Also, they serve as a first defense against the enemies as you can hide inside and wait for the right moment to attack, if necessary.

There are many methods and techniques through which you can build shelters robust enough to stand a storm. In this chapter, we are discussing two primitive types of such accommodations i.e. half-cave and fallen tree shelter. You can build on your own to fight the harsh weathers.

The Half-cave Shelter:

Shelters provide protection from the sun or rain and snow. Therefore, you only need them when the weather starts playing tricks with you. The easiest among all of the temporary shelters out there is the half-cave shelter. It has a lean-to structure. You only need to build a roof and erect walls on the sides.

Building the Roof:

Step # 01: Locating an Overhanging Cliff:

Using an over-hanging cliff for this shelter is optimal as you don't have to do much work. There are many other benefits in using over-hanging cliffs as a roof for your half-cave shelter as well. They are excellent at providing defense from the enemies as well as protection from the harsh weathers.

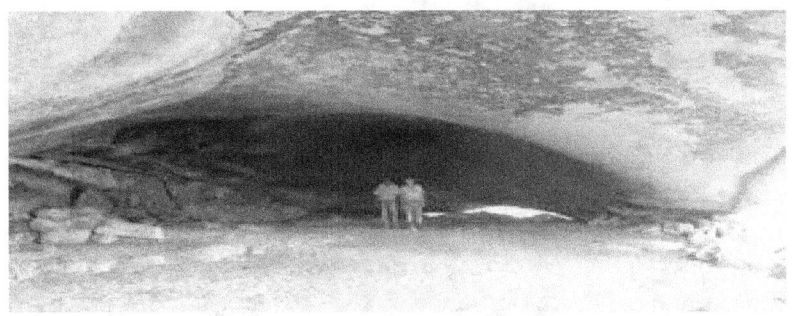

Step # 02: Finding Long Poles or Branches:

If you are unable to locate any over-hanging cliff in the current area, then you must find a pole or a stable branch of eight to ten meters in length. Secure this pole or branch to a sturdy tree at the height of your waistline. It will allow you to sit straight inside.

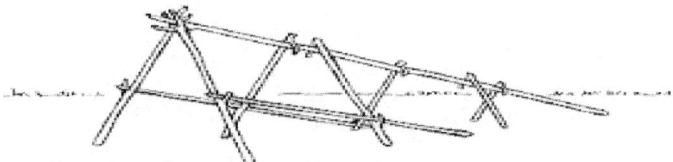

Rest the other end of the pole on the ground. Fix it in there so it does not move or slide with the wind. Add more branches on the sides to strengthen the framework. Now is the turn to build walls.

Building the Walls:

Step # 01: Collecting the Green Boughs:

Gather a few green boughs. The leaves must adhere to them. They will provide you shade from direct sunlight and also, will protect you from drizzling raindrops in the first few days of the build. Torrential rains can enter inside. Once the leaves get dry, put some fresh green boughs on the previous ones.

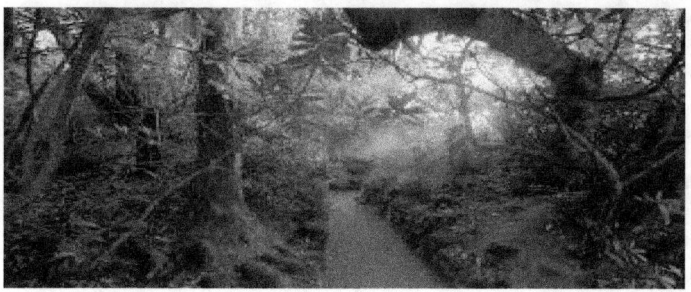

Remember that you can have some uninvited friends on these green branches such as insects and ants. But they are part of the green. You cannot get rid of them all together.

Step # 02: Resting the Green Boughs:

Rest all of the green boughs against the cliff or the pole. It is important to rest all of the boughs on their heads on the ground. Use flexible green branches to thatch the branches to build the basic framework.

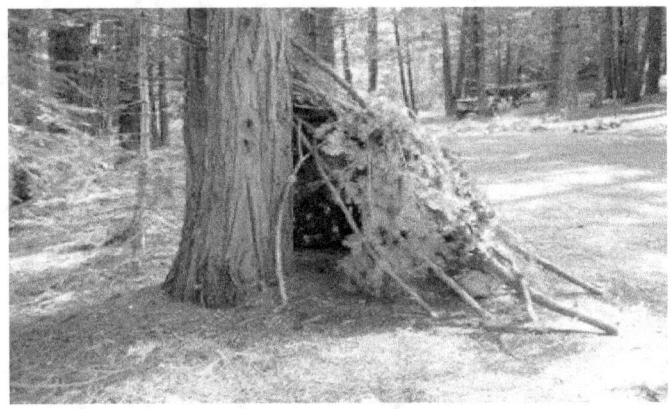

The reason for placing them this way is to steer the water to the ground. Erecting them in straight position will lever the rain drops into the shelter, and you will get no place to sit in there.

Step # 03: Camouflaging the Shelter:

No shelter made out there in the wild is safe. You can make it strong enough to stand the storms but hiding it will provide you protection and safety from both the wild animals and unfriendly passer-bys.

For camouflaging, gather some branches (both green and dried) from your immediate surroundings. Add a layer of the gathered wood on the sides and roof of your temporary accommodation. You can also add a layer of dried leaves or fill them in between the gaps of the branches to match the surroundings.

The Fallen-tree Shelter:

These temporary accommodations use less wood and have an original build. You can create them on a fallen tree by adding branches and poles on the sides to strengthen the framework and then laying layers of green boughs to provide coverage.

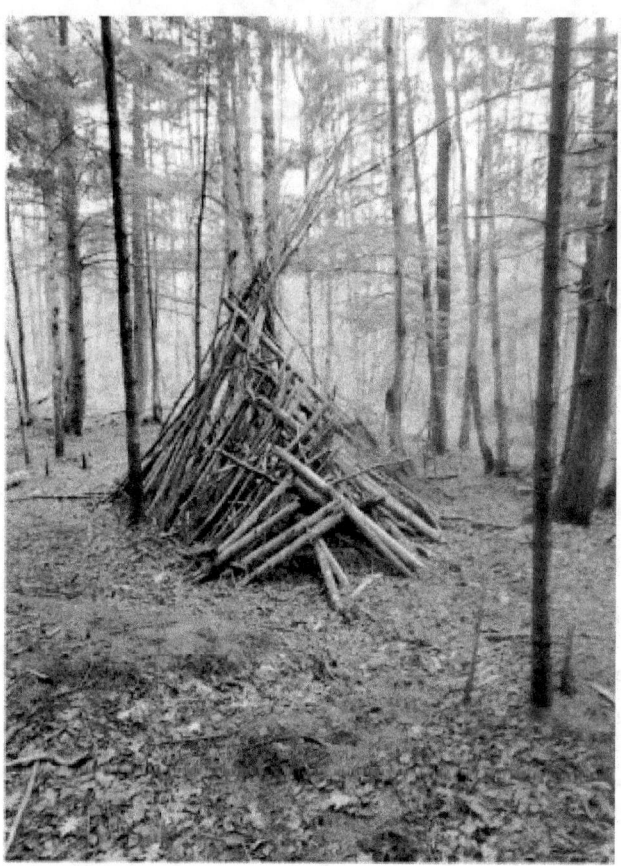

Building the Roof:

Step # 01: Locating a Fallen Tree:

The first step to building this kind of shelter is to find a fallen tree. It must be on the highest and driest ground. It must be robust enough to take the load of branches and high sufficiently to accommodate you under it.

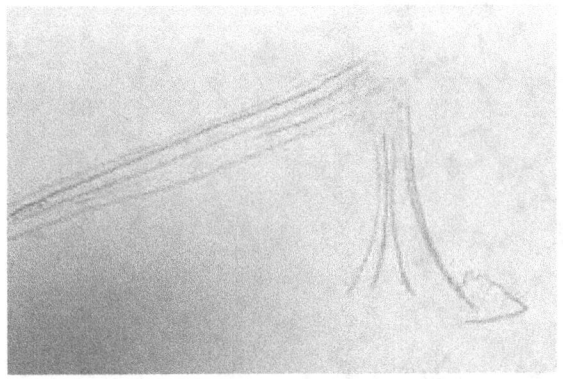

Step # 02: Cutting a Tree:

If you are unable to find a fallen tree in the surroundings, then you can cut if down yourself as well. Cut it partly through the trunk and drop it on the other side. It is pertinent to cut a tree that already has thick green branches. It will reduce the workload for you.

Building the Walls:

Step # 01: Gathering and Cutting Appropriate Boughs:

After you have found or cut a fallen tree, gather some branches. The quantity depends on upon how green is the fallen tree already. Add sturdy branches at a suitable distance from the fallen trunk to strengthen the framework.

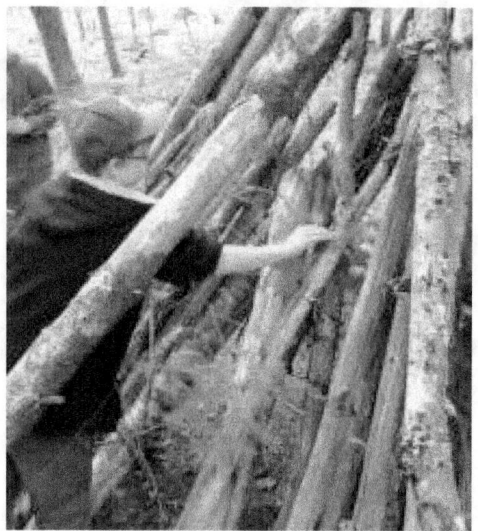

Step # 02: Secure the Branches:

After you have completed the structure, start adding small green branches in it to provide coverage. Place all the branches up-side-down. This position of the branches will steer the water to the ground. Erecting them in straight position will lever the raindrops into the shelter, and you will get no place to sit in there.

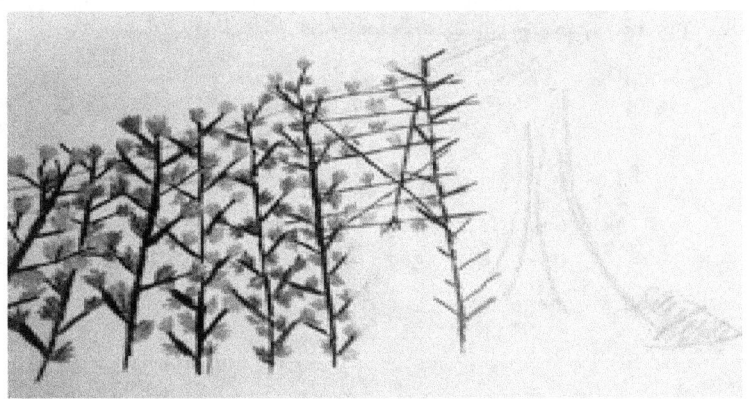

Step # 03: Camouflaging the Shelter:

Camouflaging your shelter is pertinent. It not only provides you protection from the wild animals but also helps you hide your location from the unfriendly strangers. Use branches and leaves from the immediate surroundings for camouflaging.

Chapter 03: A Frame and TeePee Shelters

It is pertinent always to plan before jumping into the process of building a shelter. The first rule of thumb to consider is to estimate the time you are going to spend in it. The Second thing is to check the weather before determining the type of shelter to build. We are discussing two types of primitive shelters for you in this chapter.

Building an A-Frame Shelter:

A-frame shelters are easy to create and provide you ample protection from the sun and rain. You can use them for extended periods. They are also easily camouflaged.

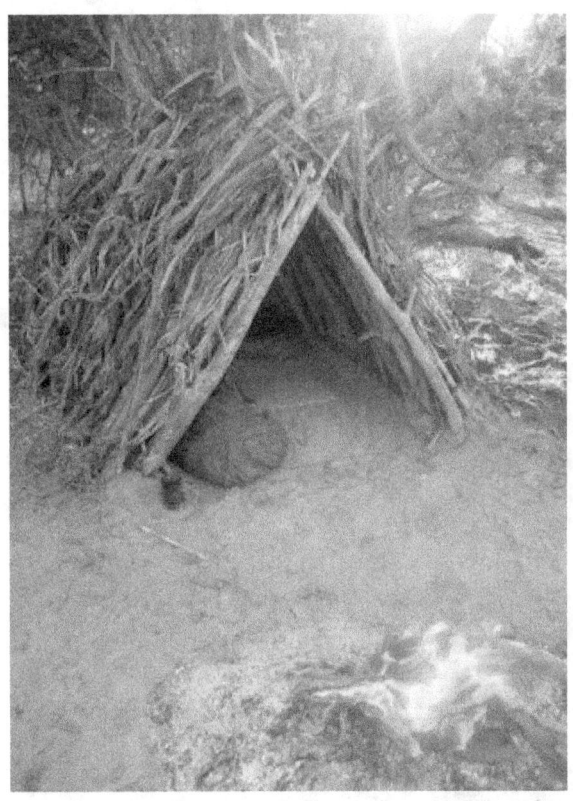

Step # 01: Finding a Location:

Choose a site to construct the A-frame shelter. It is pertinent to identify the risks before deciding the place. Stay away from the traveling rails. Also, avoid the dense area with thick trees as most of the wild animals like to inhabit in such areas.

Step # 02: Constructing the Frame:

You need one long pole to run it along the top, two small poles to make the arms of the ridgepole, sturdy branches of different sizes to make the ribs, flexible branches or rope to secure the framework and a lot of dry leaves and branches to fill the frame. Gather the wood.

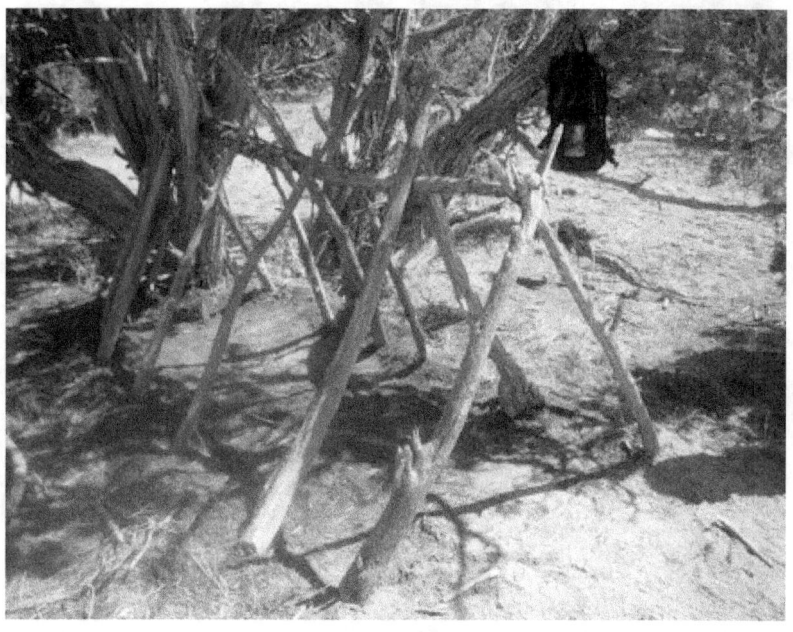

Take the longest among all poles and make it the central beam. If it is not long enough, then tie two branches together. Insert one end of this pole in the ground firmly. Take two small branches and secure them with the hanging end of the pole. Rest these arms on the ground. Add ribs to the framework.

Step # 03: Filling in the Framework:

Gather as many small green and dried branches as much thick you want your temporary house to be. Camouflaging your shelter to its surroundings is pertinent. Therefore, always pick the filling and thatching material from the immediate environment. Gather the material and fill in the gaps of the structure. There must not be any holes left in it. Also, place long green branches on their heads. It will draw the rainwater directly to the ground, and the inside area of your temporary home will not get flooded.

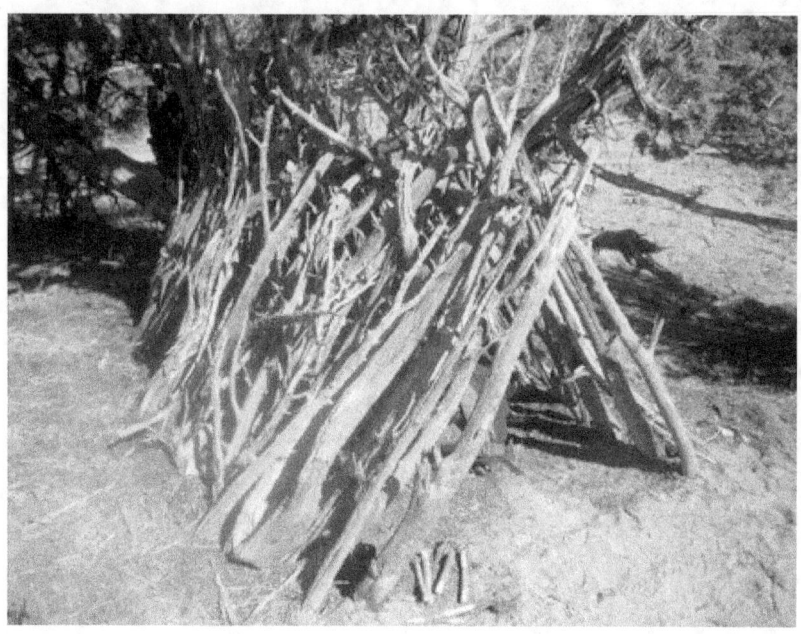

http://cdn.instructables.com/FJE/Q7WW/HUDEPJOE/
FJEQ7WWHUDEPJOE.MEDIUM.jpg

Building a Teepee Shelter:

Teepee shelters are very much like the A-frame shelters, but they provide less inner space than them. And you can make them anywhere. They are portable too.

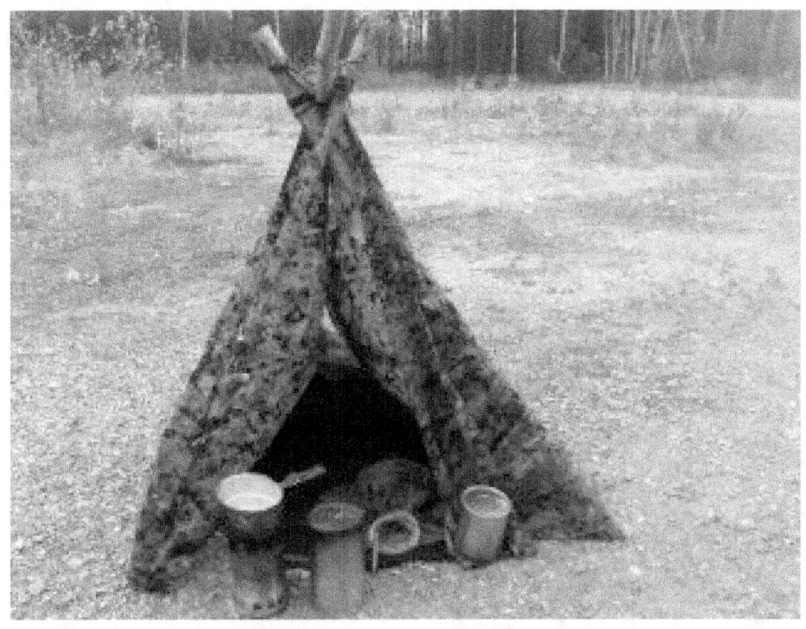

Step # 01: Picking up the Sticks:

After selecting a safe and risk-free location, probably near a natural water source, it is the time to gather sticks for your teepee shelter. Collecting right type of sticks for the framework is pertinent. Otherwise, it can result in a total loss both in terms of time and efforts. You need three main poles. One must be taller than your head. The other two must reach your height. The poles must be two to three inches wide, and the must not be broken from anywhere. If any of them is broken then first, lash it firmly before incorporating it into the framework.

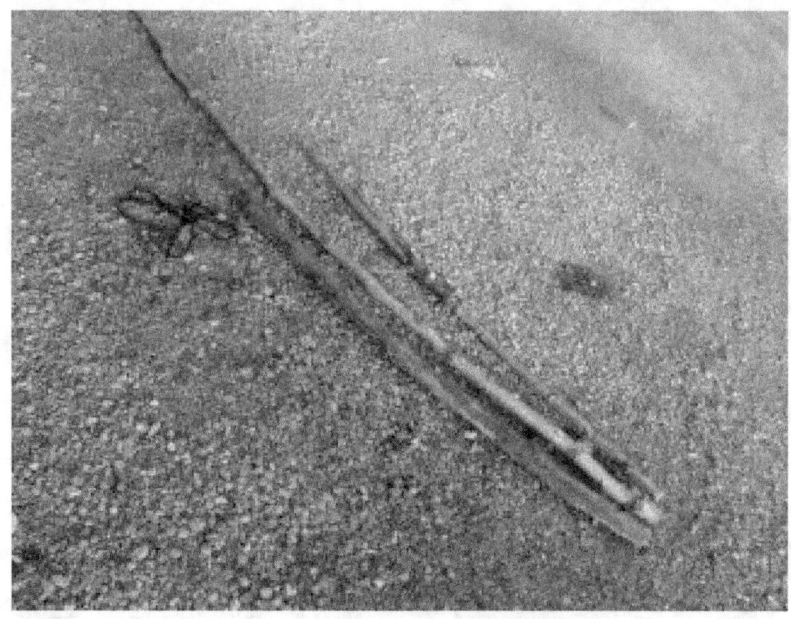

Step # 02: Lashing the Sticks Together:

Place all three of the sticks on the ground. Balance their tops. Now fasten them together firmly. Using rope or shoe laces for this purpose is ideal. But in the wild, you can also use flexible branches to tie the sticks up. Keep the knots real tight.

Step # 03: Standing the Frame up:

After you have tied them all together tightly, now stand the structure on the ground. Wedge the ends of the poles into the ground firmly. You can also place heaps of mud and small stones around the wedged poles to strengthen the framework.

Spread the arms of the structure and insert them into the ground as well. You do not need to put ribs in the frame. It is a small structure that you are going to use for sitting purposes mostly.

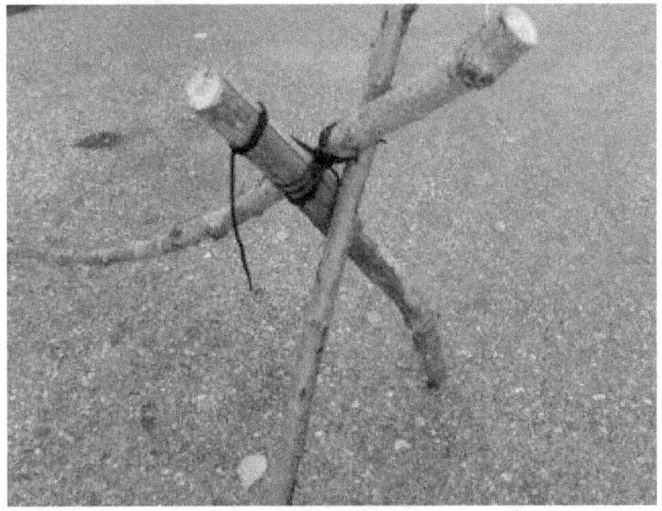

http://cdn.instructables.com/FPJ/80R2/GT9U8P2Z/ FPJ80R2GT9U8P2Z.MEDIUM.jpg

Step # 04: Covering the Framework:

After wedging the poles firmly into the ground, you are ready to cover the structure. You can use dry leaves and green branches for this purpose. Also, camouflage your shelter to the surroundings. It is helpful in providing you protection from both the wild animals and unfriendly strangers. As the shelter is all made up of wood, it is pertinent to light the fire outside your temporary accommodation.

Chapter 04: Tips to Build Indian Shelters and Shacks

Native red men of India have developed many designs and styles in temporary shelters. They are being used successfully by them for centuries. However, they come with the defects of ill ventilation and dirtiness. But they are very useful in providing shade and shelter. We are discussing various kinds of Indian shelters and shacks and the tips for building them accurately in the chapter. Let's read together!

Tips for Building Indian Navajo:

Navajo is a teepee shape shelter. Navajo Indian adopted this style in shelters to shed the rain. It is very easy to build and lasts for an extended period.

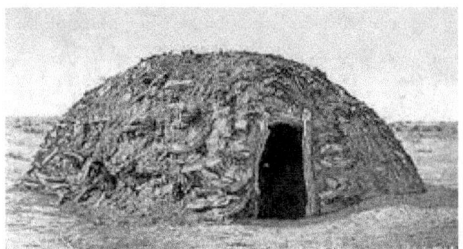

Framework: Its structure includes three forked sticks and other poles and branches. Its framework has the shape of a teepee shelter. Insert three sturdy sticks into the ground nearby in the form of a circle. Interlock the forked sticks together at the top.

Layering: Navajo Indians layer this framework with dirt. But if you are building it in the wild as a survival tool then you must use branches and leaves from the immediate surroundings to fill the structure. It will camouflage your shelter. This camouflaging helps you in hiding in the wild both from the dangerous animals and unfriendly strangers.

Tips for Building Indian Adobe Roof:

Adobe is a mixture of material for building roofs on your shelters. Straw and dirt are mixed and baked into hard bricks to make adobe roofs. Using large stones is also an option here. Yo can place them on the ceiling.

Filling the Roof: You can use sod, rushes, grass, hay, straws, dry or green leaves, and browse and small boughs to cover the poles in the wild.

Slanting the Roof: You can also slant the roof of your shelter instead of keeping it straight. Straight roofs only provide shades from the sun. A slanting roof protects you from almost any kind of climate.

Tips for Building Indian White Men's Walls:

White men keep walls of their shelters perpendicular to each other. It provides more space inside the accommodation than the other styles of temporary accommodations. But the problem here is that you cannot find suitable material to fill these walls in the wild.

Erecting Planting Walls: Therefore, erecting planting walls are more appropriate for building shelters in the wild than in the countryside. Dry leaves and green branches are used to layer these walls which are easier than the vertical ones.

Camouflaging Your Shelter: Also, this kind of walls make it easy for you to hide your refuge in the wild as it's hard to find straightly erected frameworks there. Planting walls make it very much a part of the surroundings in the wild.

Tips for Building Indian Pima Lodge:

It is an amazing style of shelter widely adopted by a majority of the Indians. The amazing quality of Pima lodge lies in adapting to the necessities of the surroundings like getting warm and tight or fresh and airy as per the climate.

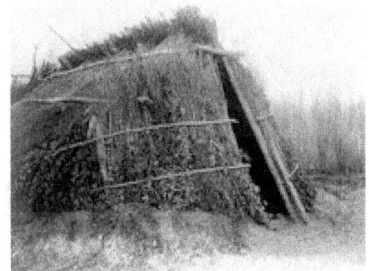

Framework: The structure of Pima lodge is like that of wick-up shelters. However, the sides of this lodge consist of leaning poles instead of the four upright posts. It makes it more adaptable to the wild surroundings. Again, it is helpful in camouflaging.

Tips for Building Indian Chippewa Shack:

Chippewa shacks are a modification of the San Carlos Apache.

Framework: These shacks have a similar dome-shaped frame like San Carlos Apache, but the layering on the structure is entirely different from that of the Apache.

Layering: Chippewa Indians use this kind of shelter mostly. They cover the structure with layers of birch bark. They are kept in place with the help of ropes. However, this practice is not possible in the wild. Therefore, you can use branches, palm leaves, palmetto leaves, straw, hay, and browse to thatch the walls. You can also plaster them with mud.

Tips for Building Indian San Carlos Shack:

San Carlos shack is a dome-shaped framework of small saplings.

Framework: You can find these young branches in the wild quickly. The ends of these branches or poles are sunk in the ground firmly in the form of a circle. You can also repeat the series by making an inner circle of these small saplings as well.

Roof: The free ends of these poles are bent and tied at the top. It gives it the shape of a dome and also provides strength and stability to the structure as the overlapping saplings are interlocked.

Layering: In the countryside, the framework is thatched with overlapping rows of bear-grass. However, in the wild, you can plaster it with mud or fill with dry leaves and green branches.

Tips for Building Indian Apache Hogan:

It is a traditional tent shape Indian shack. It has the particular framework and layering, but the difference is that rank grass instead of birch bark is used for layering this framework. You can also use corn-stalks to thatch the structure in the wild.

Building shelters are inevitable for survival in the wild and on your campsite. Indians have invented and modified several shelters and shacks over the time. However, these temporary accommodations are often ill ventilated and dirty. Both of these defects can be drawn away. You can build Windows in any of these styles by considering the element factors of the surroundings such as the kind of wild animals wandering around and the type of weather you are experiencing at that time. Else, all of these shelters are protective and have an easy built.

Chapter 05: How to build a shelter in snow

Snow shelters are made to create an insulating environment for your survival under harsh and cold weather conditions. These shelters can maintain a constant temperature of 36 degrees centigrade. Lighting a tea candle take it up to 40 degrees inside. It happens because snow is composed of trapped air. You can survive in these temporary accommodations without adequate sleeping material or clothing. Also, you don't need many tools, equipment, and materials to build these snow shelters, and you need only basic knowledge.

Step # 01: Identifying Risks:

It is pertinent to identify all kinds of risks that you can encounter at the location where you intend to build your snow shelter. Do not construct the accommodation at an area that is going to be wiped out by falling trees, falling rocks, avalanche, and landslide or similar.

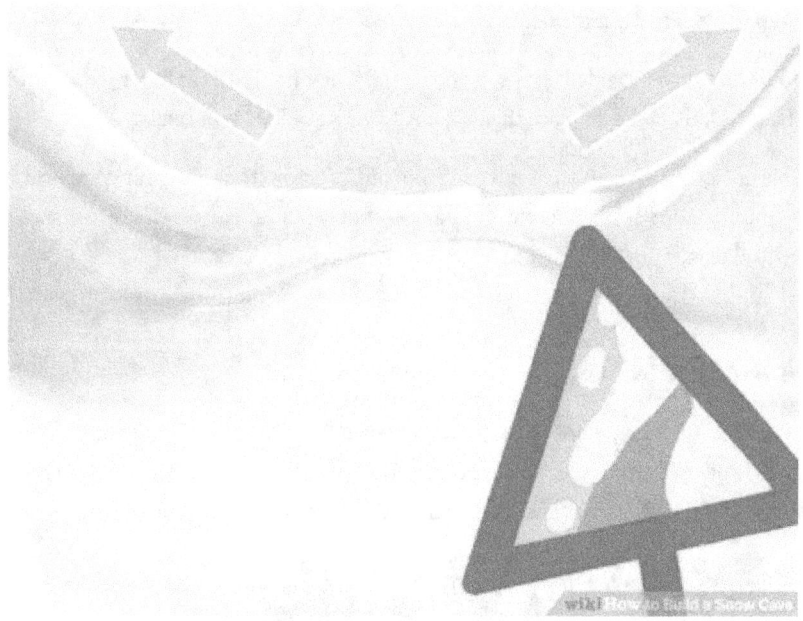

It can be difficult for you to locate your snow shelter if you leave at night or during a storm. It is recommendable to mark it with a bright color flag so you can reach it back. These flags also prevent you walking over the shelter and thus, collapsing it.

It is pertinent to poke a breathing hole in your snow shelter as carbon monoxide, and carbon dioxide can trap inside if you are lightening a candle.

The construction process is tiring, and you can sweat. Therefore, take off the insulating layers of your clothing and wear the waterproof jackets as the process can cover you in snow. Also, wear gloves to keep your hands from freezing.

Step # 02: Finding a Location:

Follow the tips provided above in your mind when finding a place for your snow shelter. Don't choose a place that is going to get you killed eventually.

You are going to need a significant amount of snow to build your temporary accommodation in it. Therefore, final a location that already has a lot of snow instead of exerting yourself out in gathering it.

Step # 03: Selecting the Type of Shelter for You:

Selecting, which type of shelter to build, depends on the location, the amount of snow, and your physiological conditions. You can build a quinzee shelter. It takes four to five hours to make as it is a hallowed out mount. It will be warm inside.

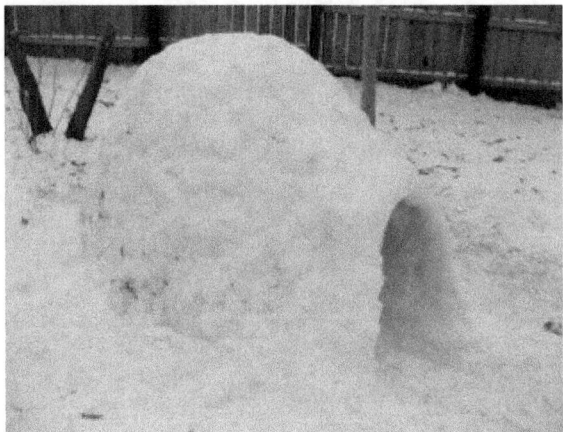

You can also dig a trench in the snow. It must be big enough to accommodate your body altogether. You can cover this trench with pine boughs, jacket, rainfly, trap, or similar. This type of shelter is just protection from the direct wind and snow. It won't be warm inside.

Step # 04: Piling Snow:

It is important when you are building a snow shelter above the ground. Gather a pile of snow of at least five to six feet height and seven to eight wide. After mounting it at a safe location, walk on it with your shoes. The snow will compress. Give it ninety minutes to two hours to settle down. It will strengthen the structure.

Step # 05: Hollowing it out:

Gather some sticks from your surroundings. They must be of eighteen inches to two feet length. Start poking these sticks in the packed snow in the form of a circle. Leave an entrance. It is ideal to keep the opening away from the wind. It will keep the insides warm.

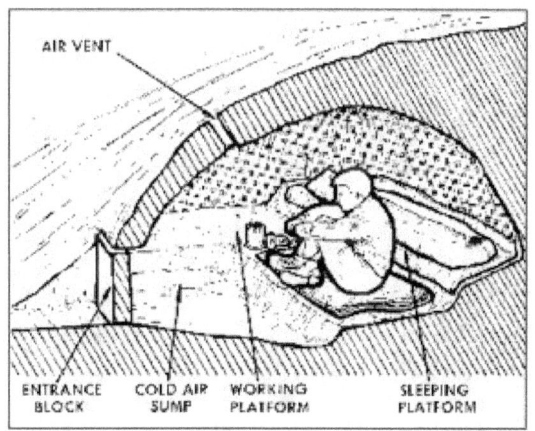

Now start digging in the snow from the center of the framework. Stop when you hit the measuring sticks forming the circle.

Step # 06: Building a Sleeping Platform:

There are two ways to create a sleeping platform within a snow shelter. The first one is to leave the sleeping area one inch higher than the ground of the shelter. Dig a trench to the entrance from under the sleeping platform. It will allow the cold air to leave the compartment as you warm it up with your body heat.

The second option is to keep the ground of the snow shelter leveled. And then build up a raised sleeping platform over it. Keep it at least one foot higher than the ground. It will help you to get the same effect on the cold air.

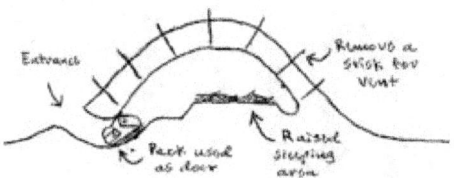

You also need to put some insulation between your body and the snow when you sleep. You can put gathered branches on your sleeping platform. You can also lay down your parachute bag and extra clothing.

Don't forget to check the breathing hole before falling asleep. Take a small branch and poke in it if it has closed by the dripping snow.

A Few Tips:

Snow naturally allows a little light to pass through it. But for lightening up the inside real bright, you need to go a few miles further. You can easily find icicles in the snowing surroundings. Gather some of them. Poke them through the roof of your temporary arrangement and they will reflect the light.

Another option is to light your candle inside a lantern or a glass jar. Then make a shelf of snow in one wall of your temporary accommodation and place it on the shelf.

It is a hustle to leave your snow shelter at night or during a snowstorm to go outside and pee. You can instead use an empty water bottle for this purpose.

If you are planning to live in the temporary accommodation for an extended period, then it is ideal to build an outdoor living area in it. It will block the cold air from entering into your sleeping compartment.

If you are lighting a candle inside, then place it on a raised platform or directly on the ground. It will keep the fire away from the melting snow.

If you want to melt the snow to convert it into drinking water, then put it in the pot with a little warm water already in it. Then heat it up on the fire.

Conclusion

Shelters are necessary to protect us from sun, rain, snow, and wind. Therefore, you only need them when the weather starts playing tricks with you. You can choose many sites to build your temporary accommodation. However, you must keep the risk factors and self-reliance opportunities of the location before finalizing one.

There are many methods and techniques through which you can build shelters robust enough to stand a storm. You can also build shelters in the wild as well as in the snow. Remember that no housing made out there in the open is safe. You can make it strong enough to stand the storms but hiding it will provide you protection and safety from both the wild animals and unfriendly passer-bys.

FREE BonusReminder

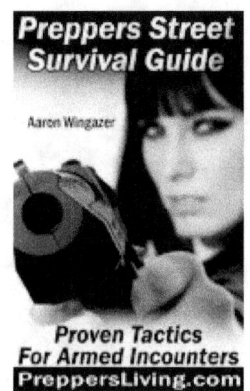

If you have not grabbed it yet, please go ahead and download your special bonus report *"DIY Projects. 13 Useful & Easy To Make DIY Projects To Save Money & Improve Your Home!"*

SimplyClicktheButtonBelow

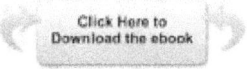

OR **Go to This Page**

http://preppersliving.com/freehttp://preppersliving.com/free

http://preppersliving.com/free

BONUS #2: More Free & Discounted Books

Do you want to receive more Free & Discounted Books?

We have a mailing list where we send out our new Books when they go free or with a discount on Kindle. Click on the link below to sign up for Free & Discount Book Promotions.

=> Sign Up for Free & Discount Book Promotions <=

OR Go to this URL

http://zbit.ly/1WBb1Ek

www.ingramcontent.com/pod-product-compliance
Lightning Source LLC
Chambersburg PA
CBHW061929280526

45787CB00004B/1535